YOGA FOR BETTER SEX

YOGA POSES AND ROUTINES FOR INCREASING SEXUAL PLEASURE AND OVERCOMING SEXUAL DYSFUNCTION

AVENTURAS DE VIAJE

Illustrated by
NEIL GERMIO

Copyright SF Nonfiction Books © 2014

www.SFNonfictionBooks.com

All Rights Reserved
No part of this document may be reproduced without written consent from the author.

WARNINGS AND DISCLAIMERS

The information in this publication is made public for reference only.

Neither the author, publisher, nor anyone else involved in the production of this publication is responsible for how the reader uses the information or the result of his/her actions.

CONTENTS

Introduction   vii

Chakras   1
Full-Stomach Breathing   2
Solo Yoga Routine   3
Partnered Yoga Routine   29
Quick Lists   41
References   44

Author Recommendations   45
About Aventuras   47

THANKS FOR YOUR PURCHASE

Did you know you can get FREE chapters of any SF Nonfiction Book you want?

https://offers.SFNonfictionBooks.com/Free-Chapters

You will also be among the first to know of FREE review copies, discount offers, bonus content, and more.

Go to:

https://offers.SFNonfictionBooks.com/Free-Chapters

Thanks again for your support.

INTRODUCTION

Yoga is amazing for sex, and is a low-impact way to maintain your body.

This routine in particular is specifically designed to:

- Increase sexual pleasure
- Alleviate sexual dysfunctions
- Intensify orgasms
- Increase sexual stamina

Even if you already have an exercise routine, you should add/include a yoga routine.

Some poses can be challenging. Adjust them to what you are capable of. Do your best and work your way up to them.

Never strain, and only remain in each position for as long as you want or as long as you feel comfortable.

CHAKRAS

Chakras are the energy centers in your body. Ideally, energy flows freely through them and in a balanced manner. When energy is not flowing freely, it leads to illness, emotional upset, etc.

The chakras are often referred to in yoga or tantric sex. From bottom to top, these are the names of the chakras and where they are located.

1st : Root/Base : Base of the spine.

2nd: Sacral : Lower abdomen.

3rd : Solar Plexus : Upper abdomen.

4th : Heart : Just above the heart.

5th : Throat : Throat

6th : Third Eye : Forehead between the eyes.

7th : Crown : Very top of the head.

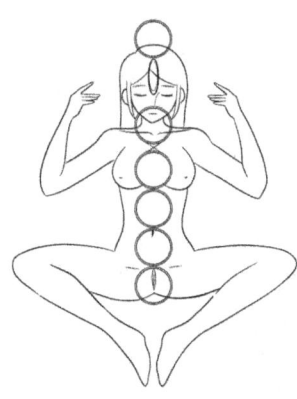

FULL-STOMACH BREATHING

Deep breathing is immensely beneficial in everyday life and an energy booster. It is also a key aspect of yoga, and is great during massage, foreplay, masturbation, and sex.

1. With your mouth closed, breathe in deeply through your nose. Count to four as you do so. Your ribs and stomach should expand as you fill up with air. As you inhale, imagine your body and chakras being filled with the clear, positive energies of love and happiness.
2. When you cannot breathe in any more, hold the breath for a count of two, then fully exhale to a count of four through your nose and/or mouth, pushing your stomach to your spine. Imagine all cloudy toxins, stress and negativity exiting your body.

Once in your pose (and while you adopt the pose), use full-stomach breathing and focus on the feelings in your chakras, especially the heart and base.

Related Chapters:

- Chakras

SOLO YOGA ROUTINE

Mountain

Stand tall, with your feet shoulder-width apart. Spread your toes wide, straighten your legs, and draw your stomach in. Lift your chest, and roll your shoulders back keeping your head in line with your shoulders.

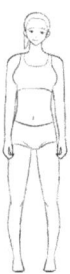

Standing Gentle Back Bend

Interlace your fingers and raise both arms over your head. Reach as high as you can. Look to your hands and bend back.

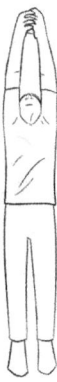

Side Bend

Drop one hand to your side and arc your other arm over your head, reaching to the side of the dropped hand. Repeat on your other side.

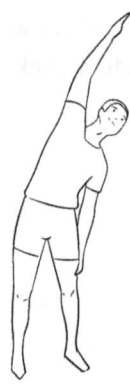

Bar-back

Keeping your legs, back and arms straight, place your hands on your thighs or knees. Roll your shoulders back and lift your head so you're looking straight ahead. Bend your knees if you need to.

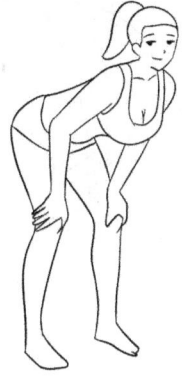

Spread-Leg Forward Bend

Stand with your feet facing forwards and approximately double shoulder-width apart. Keep your legs and back straight and bend forward at the hips. Aim to touch the floor with flat palms.

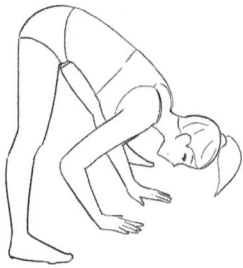

Ankle Grip

With your legs together, bend at the waist and grab the back of your calves or ankles. Keep your legs straight and pull your chest towards your knees.

AVENTURAS DE VIAJE

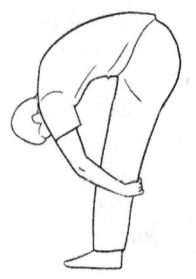

Eagle

Cross your right elbow over your left elbow and bring your left fingertips toward the base of your right palm. Bring your right leg over your left and tuck your right foot behind your left ankle. Fix your gaze to help with balance, and lift your elbows straight up toward the sky. Swap sides.

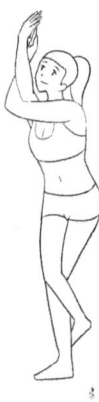

Prayer Twist

Stand with your feet together. Put your palms together as if praying. Keeping your back straight, bend at the knees and bring your left elbow to the outside of your right knee. Look up over your right shoulder. Swap sides.

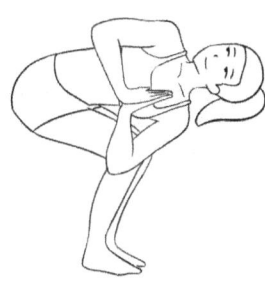

Downward Facing Dog

Get on your hands and knees, with your hands shoulder-width apart and fingers facing forwards. Keeping your arms straight, come up onto your feet. Keep your feet facing forward and shoulder-width apart. Relax your neck, straighten your legs, and press your heels down. Your final position should be an inverted V.

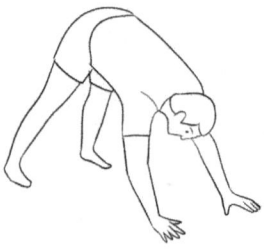

*** From Three-Legged Dog to Opener is a set which is repeated on the other side ***

Three-Legged Dog

From Downward-Facing Dog, raise your right leg as high up as you can while keeping it straight.

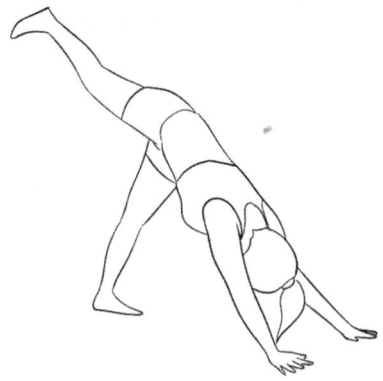

Forward Lunge

Bring your raised right leg down with your foot flat next to your right hand. Your left leg should stay straight.

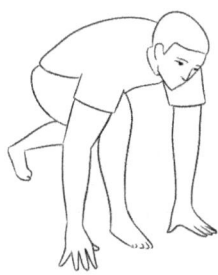

Ankle Wraps

Bring your right hand in front of your right ankle, then wrap around it counterclockwise. Your left hand should down so that you are grabbing your ankle with both hands.

When you're ready, keep your left hand wrapped around your ankle and raise your right arm to the sky. From here, drop your right hand behind your back, and clasp your hands together. Lean your head back.

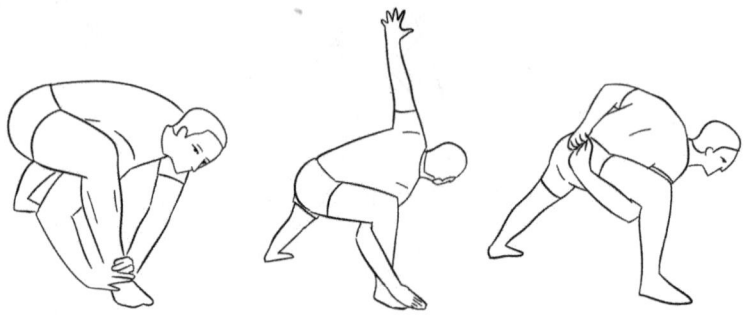

Warrior

Go back into the Forward Lunge, then straighten your back vertically and raise your hands to the sky. Look to your hands.

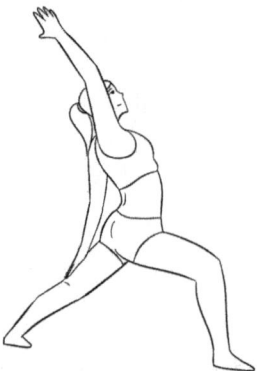

Back Lunge

Keep your right hand up and then slide your left hand down your left thigh. Your left leg should stay straight and your right leg should stay bent.

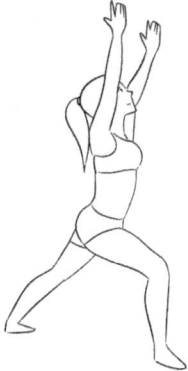

Side Twist

Go back into Warrior, then drop your right hand to the floor next to your right foot on the outside. Your left hand should go high into the air. Look up at your left hand.

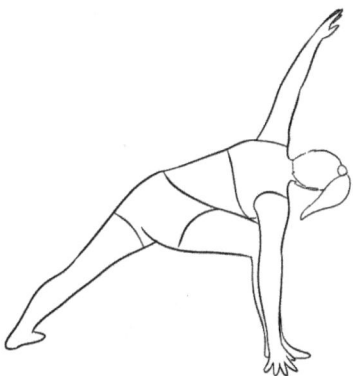

Reverse Side Twist

Go back into Warrior. Drop your left hand to the floor next on the inside of your right foot. Your right hand should go high in the air. Look to your right hand.

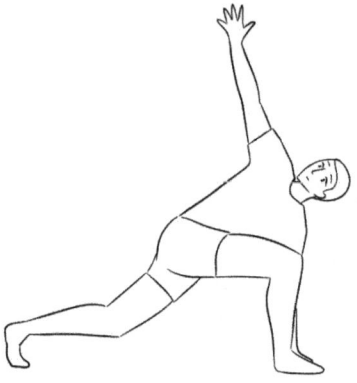

Triangle

Go back into Warrior, then straighten your right leg. Keep your left arm up and place your right hand onto your right shin. Keep your head aligned with your right foot. Look to your left hand.

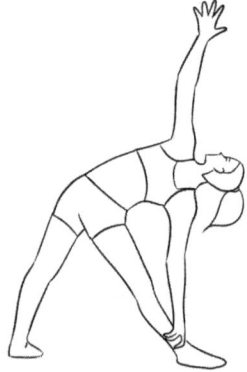

Reverse Triangle

Go back into Warrior. Keep your right hand up and reach your left arm forward to place it on your right shin. Press down on your left hand while looking up to your right hand.

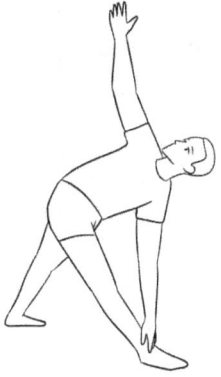

Opener

Place your hands back on the floor directly underneath your shoulders. Put your right foot close to your left hand. Lower your left knee to the floor, allowing your right knee to drop to the floor behind your right hand, so that you are on your right glute. Lift your chest, roll your shoulders back, and look up as you press your palms into the ground.

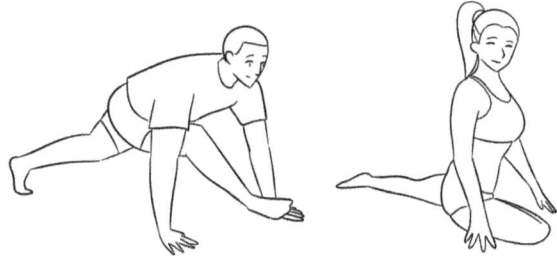

When you're ready, reach your arms forward, aiming to put your chest on the floor. Press your left hip forward and your right hip down and back.

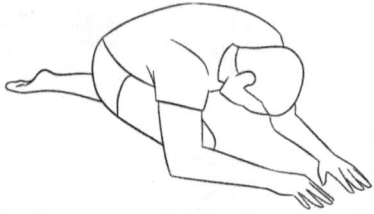

*** Repeat from Downward-Facing Dog on your left side ***

Crane

Squat down, with your feet a few inches apart. Place your hands on the floor in front of you, shoulder-width apart. Your elbows should be on the insides of your knees. Lean forward and bring your feet off the floor. Your knees should balance on your elbows. Keep the soles of your feet together.

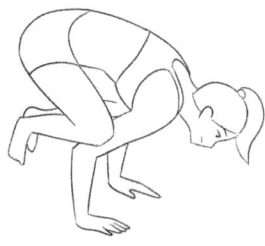

Reverse Crane

Stand straight and cross your feet. Squat down to create a gap between your knees. Place your hands on the floor, so that your elbows are on the insides of your knees with your hands on the outside of your ankles. Do not lock your elbows. Balance on your hands.

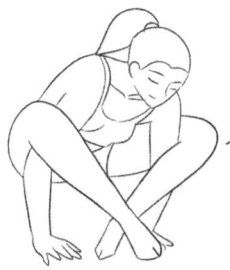

Cobra

Lie flat on your stomach, with your legs straight back and the tops of your feet on the floor. Press your palms into the floor to lift your chest. Roll your shoulders back and look up.

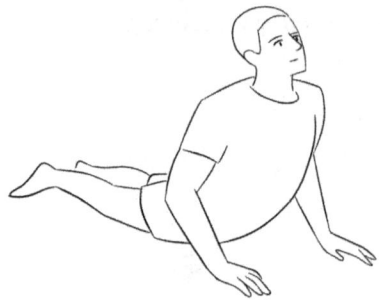

Cat Lift

Get on your hands and knees. Your hands should be directly beneath your shoulders. Look up and arch your back, pressing your stomach towards the floor.

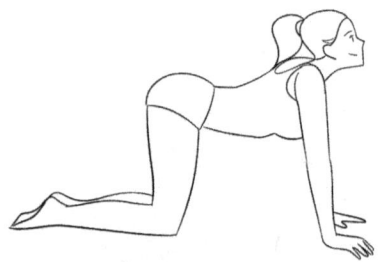

Cat Arch

Drop your head and arch your back, raising it to the sky. Suck your stomach to your spine.

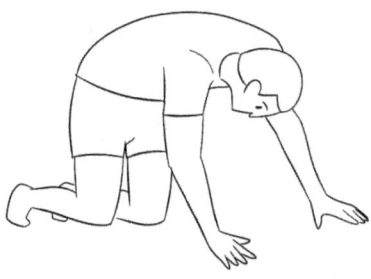

*** From Two-Legged Table to Outstretched Table is a set which is repeated on both sides ***

Two-Legged Table

Make your back level. Extend your left foot straight back and your right arm straight forward. Engage your leg and arm muscles.

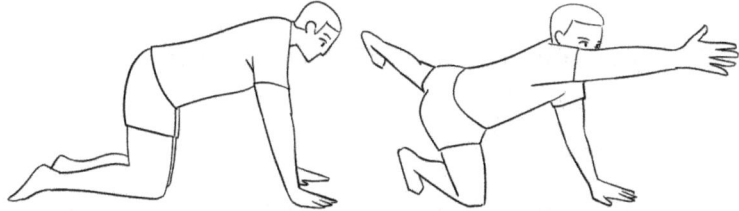

Twisted Table

Bend your left knee and grab your left ankle with your right hand.

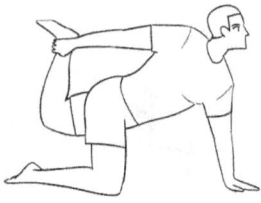

Outstretched Table

Straighten your left leg and hold it out to the left while holding your right arm straight out to your right.

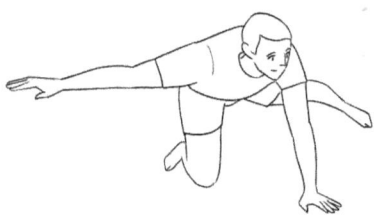

*** Repeat from Two-Legged Table on your other side ***

Forward Plank

Place your forearms flat on the floor, with your palms open and flat on the floor as well. You should be on your toes. Tighten your abdomen, back, buttocks, and legs.

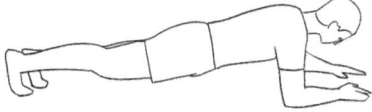

Side Planks

Lie on your side, propped up on your forearm, so that your head, torso, and feet are aligned. Your supporting elbow should be under your shoulder and in line with your hips, knees and feet.

Push up on your supporting elbow to lift your hips off the floor. Raise your arm towards the sky and look at your hand. Keep your rib cage lifted and your shoulder down.

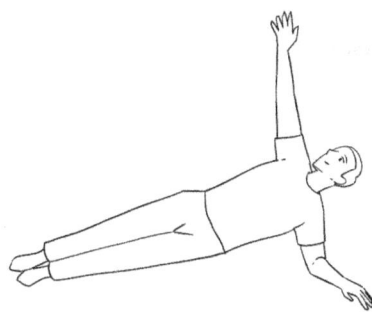

Next, support yourself on your hand instead of your forearm. Finally, raise your top leg to the sky.

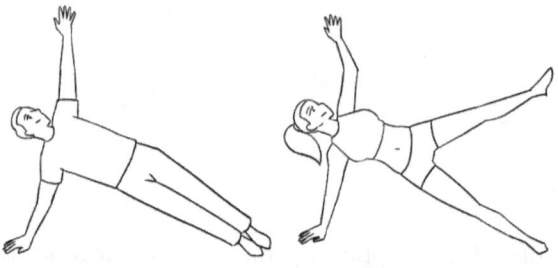

Repeat on your other side.

Frog

Lie flat on your belly. Bend your knees outwards on the floor. Prop your upper body up with your forearms. Your hands should be in a prayer position. The insides of your feet and knees should press on the floor. Bring your hips as close to the floor as possible.

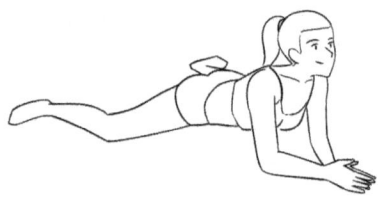

Camel

Kneel on the floor with your knees shoulder-width apart. Arch backward and grab your heels with your hands. Look behind you.

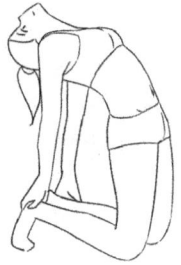

Forward Hero

Straighten your back and sit so your bum is on the floor, on the inside of your heels. Raise your arms straight above your head. Exhale and lean forward so your hands touch the floor, keeping your bum on the floor as well.

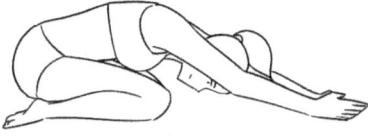

Fish

Lie on your back and put your hands under your bum. Press your forearms and elbows on the floor, lifting your upper torso and head off the floor. Rest the top of your head on the floor, but don't let it bear weight. You can also raise your feet off the floor. Keep your legs straight.

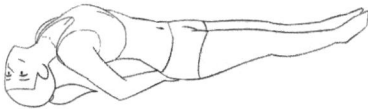

Lying-Down Leg Raises

Lie on your back and raise your leg, while keeping your other leg on the floor. With both hands, grab your leg as close to your ankle as you can and pull it towards your shoulder. Keep your legs as straight as you can. Repeat on the other side.

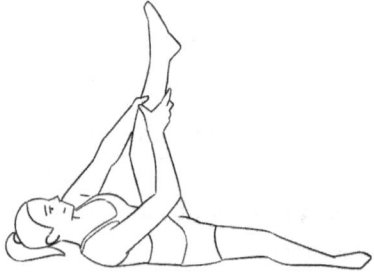

Shoulder Stand

Lie on your back, with your legs together. Keep your legs straight and roll back onto your shoulders. Use your hands on your back for support. Extend your legs and feet to the sky. Only your head, shoulders, upper arms, and elbows should touch the floor.

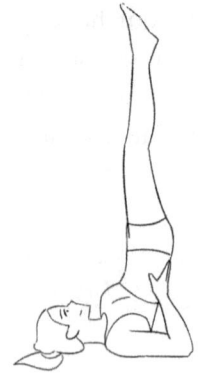

Plow

Keeping your legs straight, extend them behind your head, trying to touch your toes on the floor behind you. Lower your arms to the floor, parallel to your torso. Keep your neck off the floor by keeping your chin away from your chest.

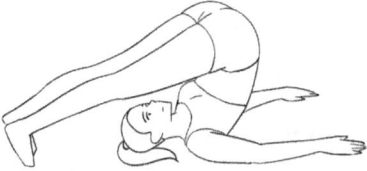

Sleeping Angel

With your feet in the air and your legs straight, spread your legs and grab your big toes. Keep your neck off the floor.

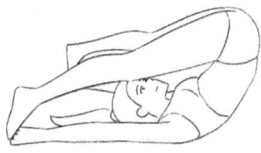

Dead Bug

Lie flat on your back and bring your knees up so the soles of your feet face the sky. With your elbows on the inside of your knees, grab the outside of each foot. Pull your knees toward the floor.

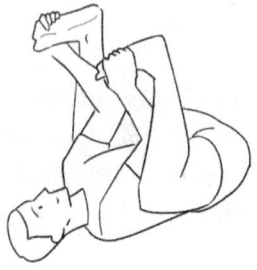

Lying Twist

Extend your arms to your sides and let your knees drop to the right while you look over your left shoulder. Cross your right ankle over your left knee and use it to press your left knee towards the floor.

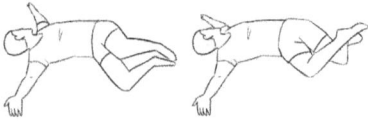

Knee Pull

With your right ankle still crossed over your left knee, grab your left knee and pull it to your chest. Relax your neck and shoulders and let your tailbone sink to the floor.

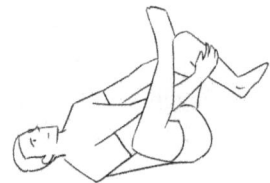

*** Repeat Lying Twist and Knee Pull on your other side ***

Bridges

If you are on hard ground, use something to provide padding for your head, such as a folded towel.

Lie on your back, with your arms parallel to your body. Bend your knees so your feet are flat on the floor. Keeping your head, neck, arms and shoulders on the floor, push with your legs and arch your back to lift your stomach to the sky.

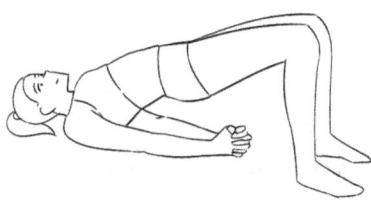

Next, place your hands flat on either side of your head. Place your feet on the ground and use them to push yourself into an arched back position, rolling on your head. Attempt to touch your nose to the floor.

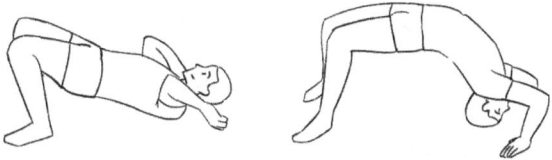

Finally, push up on your hands to raise your head off the floor.

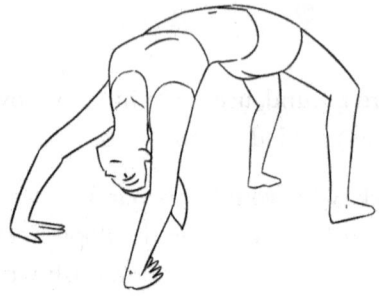

Forward Fold

Sit on the floor with your back straight and your legs straight out in front of you. Your feet should be together, with your toes pointing to the sky. Reach for your toes and pull your chest to your knees.

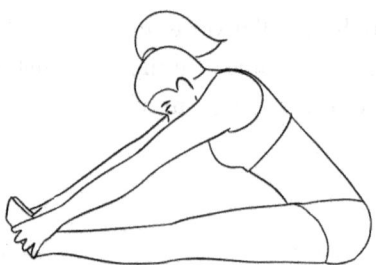

Seated Open Angel

Spread your legs as far as you can. Grab your big toes with the first two fingers of each hand. Keep your back straight and press your hips forward.

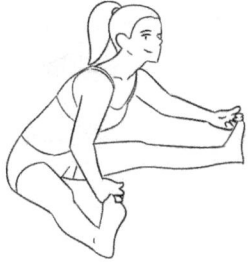

Seated Angel

Sit back up and bring the soles of your feet together. Interlock your fingers around your two big toes. Bring your feet as close to your body as possible. Keep your back straight and relax your knees toward the floor.

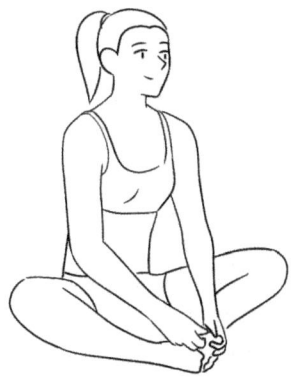

Supine Angel

Lie on your back while keeping the soles of your feet together. Rest your hands on your lower abdomen.

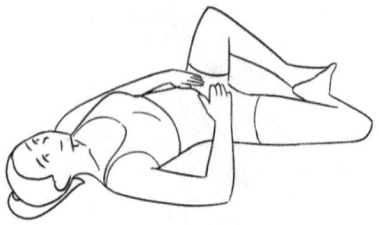

Corpse Pose

Straighten your legs, pin your shoulders to the floor, and let your hands fall by your sides, palms facing up. Concentrate on deep stomach breathing or do any other meditation you like.

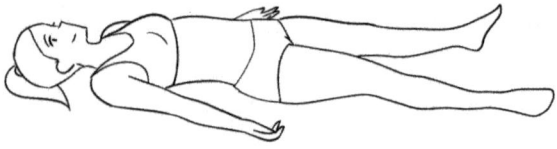

PARTNERED YOGA ROUTINE

Any method of exercising together helps to create a deeper connection. This is especially true with partnered yoga, where you will often breathe in sync and feel/concentrate on each other's energy.

If you are feeling a bit friskier, you can do the poses naked and see how far you can get before losing control. After all, many of them are taken straight from the Kama Sutra.

The poses are presented in a particular order which you can follow, but feel free to do what you wish.

Note: Many of these descriptions refer back to poses from the Solo Yoga Routine chapter.

Driving the Peg Home

Stand facing each other, bodies touching. Grab each other around the waist and use each other as support. Both arch back.

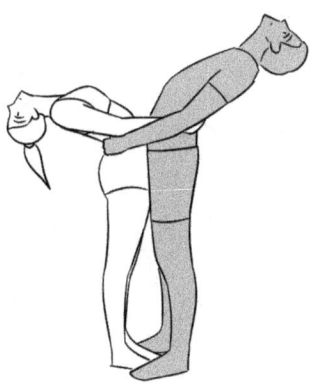

Lovers Pelvis Press

Stand facing each other, feet shoulder-width apart and about a foot away from each other. Both arch back with your hands high in the air, pressing your groins together for support.

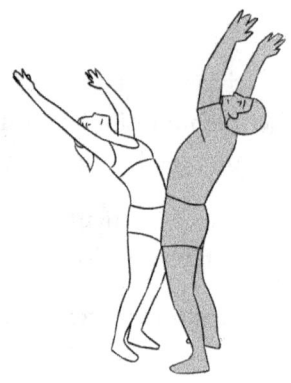

Dangling Lovers

Stand facing each other, hands together. Step apart while letting your upper torsos dangle to the floor. Keep your legs straight, with your hands meeting in the center between you.

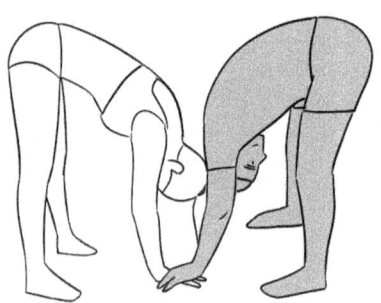

Squat-to-Stand Support

Squat down while facing each other. Hold each other's wrists and keep your backs straight. Support each other as you stand up together.

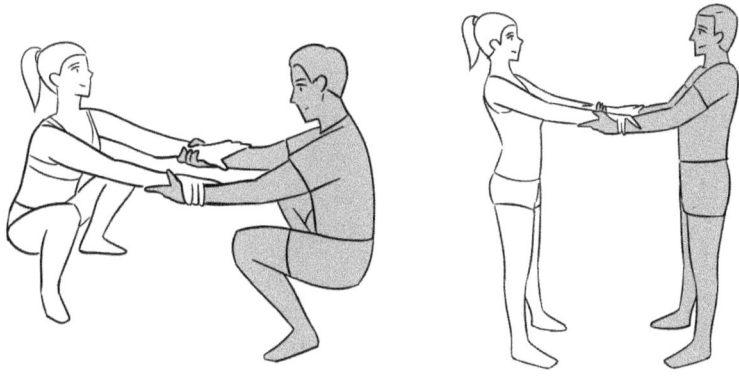

Seated Open Angels

You are both in a modified Seated Open Angel. Get close enough so your feet are touching and grab each other's wrists. Lean back to help stretch your partner stretch forward, then vice versa.

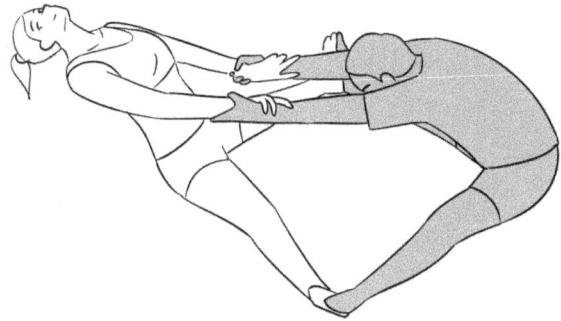

Raised Seated Open Angels

Sit as if in Seated Open Angels, but with your legs not stretched out as far. Hold hands on the outside of your legs and bring your legs up.

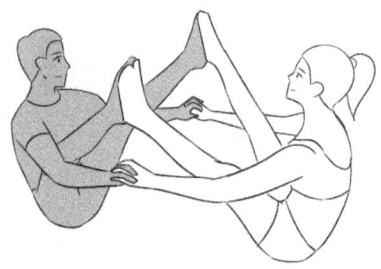

Cobras

Lie flat on your stomachs with your heads touching. With your hands under your shoulders, push your bodies up, arching your backs and looking to the sky.

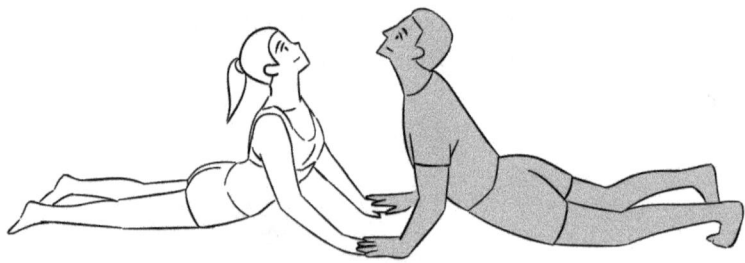

Kama's Wheel

Sit in Seated Angel. Your partner should sit in front of you, also in Seated Angel, and up against your groin. Wrap your arms around your partner and hold their ankles while they hold your feet.

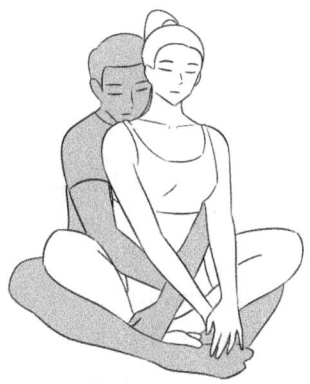

White Tiger Tao

Your partner adopts Frog. Come from behind, with your legs in Frog on top of them. Your legs should alternate, and your groin should press against your partner. Support your weight on your hands, which should be placed on either side of your partner's hips.

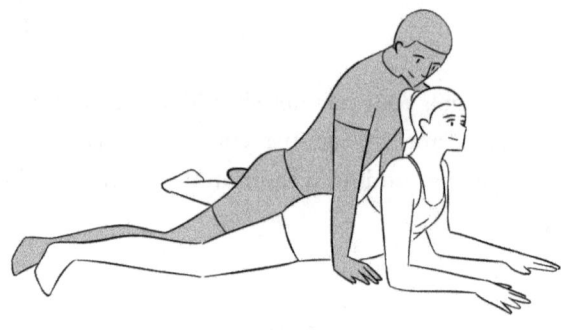

Congress of the Cow

Your partner is on their hands and knees. Their knees are shoulder-width apart under her hips, and her hands are directly underneath her shoulders. Her arms are straight. She arches her back, pushing her stomach out whilst looking up to the sky. Get behind her on your knees and press your groin against hers. Place your knees between her legs. Go into an improvised Camel, using her feet as support.

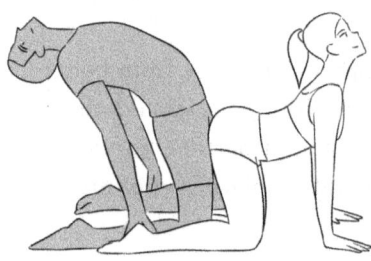

Lovers Embrace

Your partner adopts the Forward Hero. Kneel close behind her, one knee on either side of her body. Leans over her, pressing his body against hers. Positions can be swapped.

Yoga For Better Sex

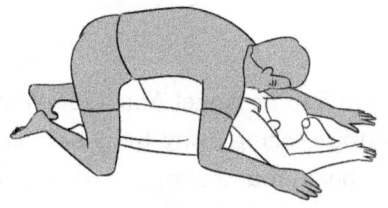

Mill Vanes

Your partner lies in Supine Angel. You adopt a modified Frog on top of them. You are facing away from her, with your legs on either side of her body. You use your hands for support, and rest your groin against theirs. Their hands rest on your bum.

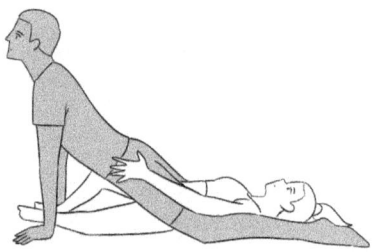

Amazon

You lie on your back and bring your knees to your chest. Your partner faces you, and you hold hands. Their feet are on either side of your hips and your legs are on either side of their torso. They squat down, bringing their groin to yours.

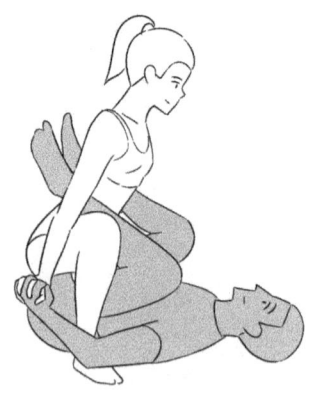

Ascending

You adopt Fish. Your partner places their knees on either side of you, so that their groin is on yours. Their hands rest on their calves, and their head on your chest.

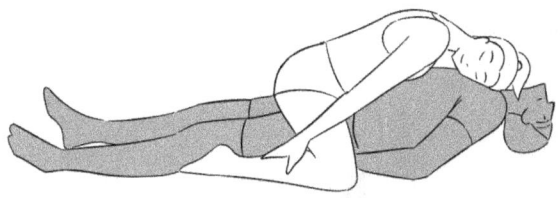

Arc

Your partner goes into the Bridge. You kneel between their legs, pressing your groin against theirs. You support them at the small of their back while they come up on the top of their shoulders. Their hands rest on your calves.

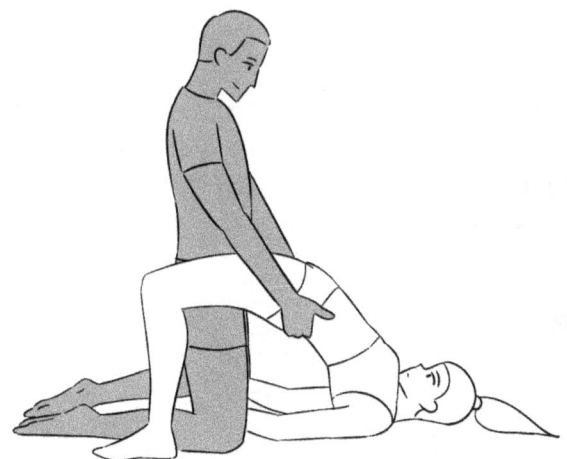

Anango-Rango

You squat with your feet double shoulder-width apart. Your partner does a back bend in such a way that their legs are on either side of your waist. Their hands are on the floor in front of you, fingers facing back towards you and eyes forward, away from you. Their legs dangle over your thighs.

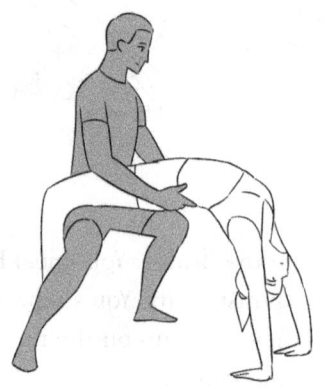

Twining

You partner performs a lying down leg raise with their left leg in the air. You face her and brings your left leg beyond their head on their right side. Your right leg stretches back on the inside of their right leg. Your groins are pressed together.

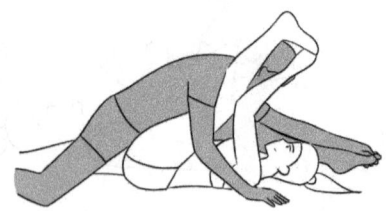

Wife of Indra

Your partner adopts Plow while you take up Camel. You touch at your groins. Your partner holds you by the back of your thighs.

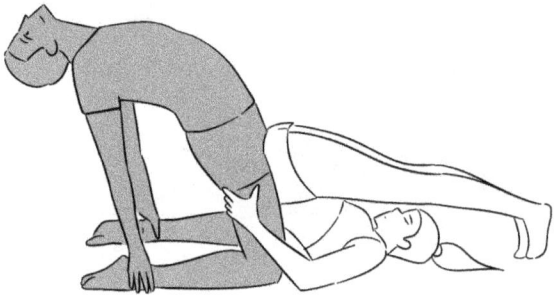

Clasping

Your partner lies on their back with their legs spread. You put your groin to theirs, keeping your body straight and supporting your weight on your toes and hands. You partner crosses their ankles around your waist. You press your hips down, pushing your upper body up off the floor at the same time.

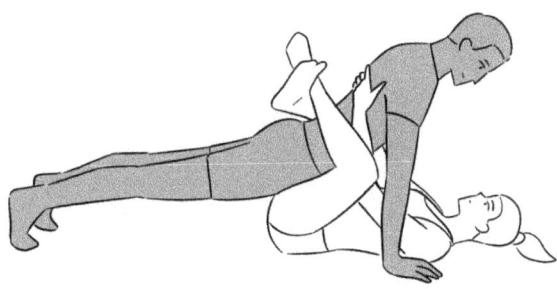

Face to Face

Your partner lies flat on their back, legs spread. You lie on top of them. Your groin rests on theirs. Your legs are straight and your feet are together. You support your weight on your toes. You and your partner grab each other's hands. You push down with your hips while lifting your upper body.

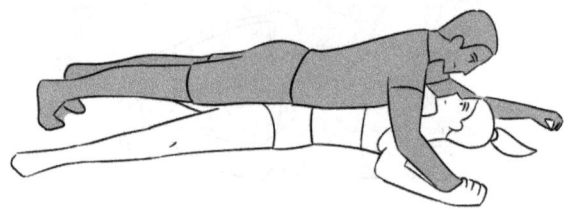

Related Chapters:

- Solo Yoga Routine

SOLO YOGA ROUTINE QUICK LIST

Mountain	Cat Arch
Standing Gentle Back Bend	Two Legged Table
Side Bend	Twisted Table
Bar-back	Outstretched Table
Spread Leg Forward Bend	Forward Plank
Ankle Grip	Side Planks
Eagle	Frog
Prayer Twist	Camel
Downward Facing Dog	Forward Hero
Three Legged Dog	Fish
Forward Lunge	Lying Down Leg Raises
Ankle Wraps	Shoulder Stand
Warrior	Plow
Back Lunge	Sleeping Angel
Side Twist	Dead Bug
Reverse Side Twist	Lying Twist
Triangle	Knee Pull
Reverse Triangle	Bridges
Opener	Sitting Stretch
Crane	Seated Open Angel
Reverse Crane	Seated Angel
Cobra	Supine Angel
Cat Lift	Dead Man

PARTNERED YOGA ROUTINE QUICK LIST

- Driving the Peg Home
- Lovers Pelvis Press
- Dangling Lovers
- Squat to Stand Support
- Seated Open Angels
- Raised Seated Open Angels
- Cobras
- Kama's Wheel
- White Tiger Tao
- Congress of the Cow
- Lovers Embrace
- Mill Vanes
- Amazon
- Ascending
- Arc
- Anango-Rango
- Twining
- Wife of Indra
- Clasping
- Face to Face

THANKS FOR READING

Dear reader,

Thank you for reading *Yoga For Better Sex*.

If you enjoyed this book, please leave a review where you bought it. It helps more than most people think.

Don't forget your FREE book chapters!

You will also be among the first to know of FREE review copies, discount offers, bonus content, and more.

Go to:

https://offers.SFNonfictionBooks.com/Free-Chapters

Thanks again for your support.

REFERENCES

DK Publishing. (2011). *Yoga for a New You*. DK

Gibbs, B. Hall, D. Smith, J.(2013). *The Complete Guide To Yoga: The essential guide to yoga for all the family with 800 step-by-step practical photographs* . Southwater.

Greaux, J. Langheld J. (2007). *Better Sex Through Yoga: Easy Routines to Boost Your Sex Drive, Enhance Physical Pleasure, and Spice Up Your Bedroom Life.* Harmony.

Lalvani, V. (2002). *Yoga for Sex: Improve Your Sex Life the Tantric Way.* Bounty Books.

Miller, O. (2004). *Essential Yoga: An Illustrated Guide to Over 100 Yoga Poses and Meditations.* Chronicle Books.

Nerve.com. (2003). *Position of the Day: Sex Every Day in Every Way.* Chronicle Books.

Vatsyayana. (2012).*The Kamasutra.* YogaVidya.com.

AUTHOR RECOMMENDATIONS

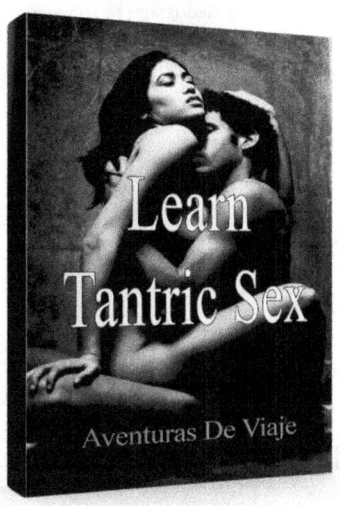

Teach Yourself Tantric Sex

Start feeling pleasure like you never have before, because this is the biggest sexual awakening you'll ever have.

Get it now.

www.SFNonfictionBooks.com/Learn-Tantric-Sex

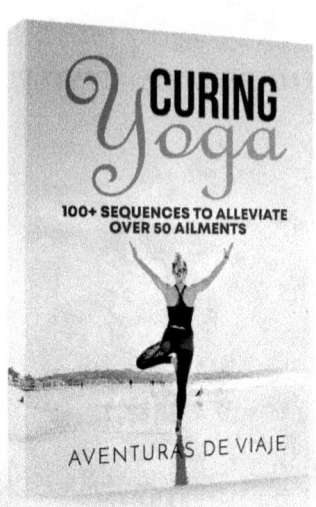

Discover How to Use Yoga as Medicine

Add this book to your collection, because with it you can use yoga to heal your mind, body, and spirit.

Get it now.

www.SFNonfictionBooks.com/Curing-Yoga

ABOUT AVENTURAS

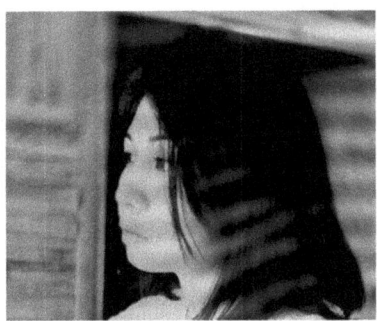

Aventuras has three passions: travel, writing, and self-improvement. She is also blessed (or cursed) with an insatiable thirst for general knowledge.

Combining these things, Miss Viaje spends her time exploring the world and learning. She takes what she discovers and shares it through her books.

www.SFNonfictionBooks.com

- amazon.com/author/aventuras
- goodreads.com/AventurasDeViaje
- facebook.com/AuthorAventuras
- instagram.com/AuthorAventuras

www.ingramcontent.com/pod-product-compliance
Lightning Source LLC
Chambersburg PA
CBHW070036040426
42333CB00040B/1691